CONTENTS

INTRODUCTION

For years our kind has wondered what makes us who we are. The question of where our personalities, latent abilities, and interests originate continues to be a question people debate even today. Many people, even those not particularly religious, point to the soul. According to Britannica.com, the soul has been classified by religion and philosophy as "the immaterial aspect or essence of a human being, that which confers individuality and humanity, often considered to be synonymous with the mind or the self." This aspect of our selves was touted as the origin of our personalities, our creativity, and our individual beliefs. It was the framework the brain worked around to control the action of the body. The concept of a soul has been around for more than a millennium, seemingly as old as time itself, used to explain why we are different from the stalwart oak or the fleeting deer.

However, as science progressed a new term for what others might consider the soul emerged: consciousness. According to Boris Kotchoubey, a professor at the Institute of Medical Psychology and Behavioral Neurobiology, "Consciousness is not a process in the brain but a kind of behavior that, of course, is controlled by the brain like any other behavior. Human consciousness emerges on the interface between three components of animal behavior: communication, play, and the use of tools." This theory relies heavily on the mind, rather than the existence of an ethereal bodily component, as did many scientific theories. The fact of the matter is, there is no way to completely prove the soul's existence. It's unquantifiable; a mere notion of something that we have no clue how to explore. The brain on the other hand is solid, composed of matter with a definite connection to the rest of the body's processes. It's something science can study and explore, the closest thing to a soul that we can analyze fully.

However, there are many people who still question if the brain is enough to shape our entire being. Are we perhaps missing a pivotal piece of the puzzle? Are our biological processes alone enough to shape our personalities, our identities? If there is a spirit, what comprises it? How do we decode and quantify the spiritual intricacies within ourselves if they remain elusive from both science and philosophy? Religious leaders, scientists, and philosophers alike have spent centuries postulating the intricacies of our human consciousness. Yet after all those years of speculation and theorizing, the concept of a soul remains like the air around us: something we can vaguely feel, but never grasp.

As an exercise, let's delve into one of these older theories. One that spans throughout time and is still thought of highly today. And that is the idea that our entire beings are comprised of a series of parts, all working together in tandem. The body, mind, and spirit: all intertwined within, each unable to work without the other. The components of who we are cannot be delegated to one of these processes, but to a combination of all of them. There cannot be one without the other. This is the sentiment that encompasses the practice of Ayurveda.

Ayurveda is a form of Traditional Indian Medicine that has been practiced for centuries, aiming not only to heal a person physically, but mentally and spiritually as well. Though its origins are deeply rooted in Hinduism, it's not simply a religious or spiritual belief, but a way of life. This practice encompasses aspects of religion, philosophy, and herbalism, and is centered around the idea that the human body and human consciousness are connected.

How we treat our consciousness has a profound effect on the body as improper care of the spirit can result in stress in a person's physical and mental health. Although skeptics might call into question the validity of Ayurvedic treatments in the medical sphere, the connection between the mind and body is something that science has proven time and time again. The problems within the mind become the problems of the body, as we have seen in patients with excess stress, depression, and paranoia.

When alternative forms of medicine are mentioned, there are normally two vastly different mindsets people gravitate towards: skepticism and optimism. Many people are skeptical about the abilities of alternative forms of medicine because of their lack of basis in science. The placebo effect is often blamed for any results that people might feel after these kinds of treatments. Persuasion can be a powerful tool; sometimes when a person is told that their condition will be alleviated, their body's inner workings fill in the gaps. Other people are skeptical of alternative forms of medicine simply because of the sheer number of charlatans surrounding this practice. For centuries, these people have taken advantage of the more naïve members of society in order to make a profit. It's understandable how these people might be cynical about the abilities of these untested alternative forms of medicine.

However, there are some people who are naturally drawn towards these ancient methods. While modern medicine has done a lot for society, it does come with its drawbacks. Cost is one of them; the need for some people to have a constant supply of medication comes with a hefty price tag. This can put a hole in a person's funds that might not have to be there if they can rely on another form of treatment. The other factor that leads people to alternative medicine is their cynicism towards pharmaceutical drugs. While vaccines and medications are a lifesaving feature of modern medicine, there have been some bad options touted by medical professionals. One only has to look at the opioid crisis of 2019 to find that sometimes certain drugs can only make a person's situation worse.

Let me just make this clear: it is not a good idea to completely remove modern medicine from the equation, isolate yourself in the mountains, and completely rely on energy healing for all your health needs. Whether we like it or not, the only reason that we are able to live for 80+ years is because of the advancements we've made in our understanding of health and medicine. Alternative forms of medicine should be complementary to the treatments we receive from our doctors, not a substitution.

That said, it couldn't hurt to incorporate Ayurveda into your routine. While some people may question the ability of some Ayurvedic treatments to heal certain diseases, the core components of the practice foster a healthy lifestyle and fulfilling view of the self and the soul. Ayurveda understands that the needs of the body reflect the needs of the mind and soul, and that's a mindset that we can attribute to everything in our lives.

THE ORIGINS OF AYURVEDA

Before we talk about what exactly Ayurveda is, it's important to understand where it came from. As many of us are aware, how we are raised and how the people around us are raised has a subconscious effect on our thought processes. For that reason, our cultures have a substantial role in shaping our behaviors, our values, and our spiritual beliefs. For this alternative form of medicine, its humble beginnings originated in ancient India. It was around this time that India had developed a series of sacred texts known as the Vedas.

These doctrines began as oral teachings, being passed down by religious leaders to educate the masses before their progression to sacred text. According to the National Ayurvedic Medical Association, "the Vedas celebrate the elements of life, especially fire, wind, and water, as well as Mother Earth and the plants and animals who dwell upon her." For many cultures during this timeframe, there was often very little separating religion from everyday life, and for India it was no different. Hinduism wasn't simply a form of worship, but a way of life, and the Vedas reflected that. The Vedas not only spoke on religious matters, but also matters involving government, sciences, and music. They were a guide dictating how to live a healthy and happy life. These texts wove these topics together with Hindu practices and beliefs, allowing the people to better understand what they learned from their religion and apply it to their lives.

Ayurveda is considered to be a subcategory of the *Vedas*, a sacred document focused on health and medicine. According to *Complementary and Alternative Medicine for Older Adults: A Guide to Holistic Approaches to Healthy Aging,* Ayurveda found its roots in these ancient Vedic texts. Its origins can be traced to the Upaveda and Atharvaveda disciplines, which dealt with applying religious knowledge for the benefits of a person's everyday life. During this time, the *Vedas* were not simply considered religious texts, but the scientific study of all life. The term Ayurveda is a combination of the Sanskrit words for life (ayur) and knowledge or science (veda), the full word translates to "knowledge of life." These Ayurvedic practices and treatments became widespread during the Bronze Age—roughly around 3000-1300 BCE—the first recorded instances of these practices being used in the lands that would later become modern-day Pakistan. These practices were a natural system of medicine that helps people understand themselves and achieve vitality within the laws of nature. Most importantly, it was something people could do on their own, allowing them to have autonomy over their own health and wellbeing.

WHAT IS A HEALTHY LIFE?

But what exactly did these texts teach people about healthy and holistic living? According to Ayusante.com, a healthy life from the perspective of Ayurveda is "One that is devoid of any physical, mental or emotional disturbance; One where the sensory perceptions are fully functional; One where Ojas (Vitality), Tejas (Shine) and Prana (Energy) are at their optimum; One where the person can perform all duties towards himself/herself, his/her family and the society without any obstacles; One where the person possess all virtues and is respected in his/her community; One where the person is happy and has attained physical, mental, emotional and spiritual peace."

These texts preached balance in a person's life, in their dosha, and in soul. Once balance was attained, the person would be capable of living their life to their full potential, without being weighed down by their inherent flaws. This was achieved by two things: preventative measures and curative measures. Even back then, people realized that the best way to keep themselves healthy was to prevent health complications before they started. In Ayurveda, this involved building good health habits, strengthening the immune system, and engaging in meditation to routinely purge the mind of stress and anxiety. These efforts were performed religiously by practitioners of Ayurveda, sculpting their lives around these methods to ensure their physical, mental, and spiritual health.

However, practitioners didn't only take care of their own bodies. They also tended to the needs of those who came to them with a variety of health complications. This is where the curative measures were usually performed. These people didn't always lead the lifestyle of Ayurveda, so they often came in hopes of being cured by them. Practitioners would often recommend various herbs and infusions to alleviate symptoms, as well as providing massages and other forms of therapy to nurse them back to health. After they finished, they would give the patient recommendations on how to prevent these diseases from popping back up. This form of medicine became a huge part of the lives of people in India, ultimately becoming an integral part of their culture.

THE EXPANSION OF AYURVEDA

These doctrines wouldn't simply stay put in the Indian subcontinent. The lands of the Indus Valley were rich and fertile, resulting in an abundance of herbs and spices. These luxuries prompted many countries to travel there in search of trade, and with the arrival of these traders came the spread of the concept of Ayurveda into Europe. The popularity of the Ayurvedic lifestyle would only grow as time went on. Now in the modern day, these teachings have experienced a resurgence, alternative forms of medicine becoming more and more appealing to western cultures.

Perhaps out of cynicism of the effect of modern medicine on the body or the hefty cost that comes with many prescription drugs, many people have been gravitating to other less expensive ways to heal their bodies and minds. Herbalists, massage therapists, and beauty gurus have made the choice to add Ayurvedic treatments to their repertoire, adopting many of the beliefs written in those ancient texts. In our internet age, the spread of these practices has spanned across the globe, amassing a new set of followers interested in getting in touch with their spiritual side.

PRAKRITI, DOSHAS, AND THE FIVE GREAT ELEMENTS

The question still stands: what is it about Ayurveda that has allowed it to retain its popularity after centuries of development in modern medicine. At the end of the day, it all comes down to its holistic approach to health. The main theme within Ayurvedic practices is that spirituality is intertwined with our minds and bodies. According to John Hopkins Medicine, "The concepts of universal interconnectedness, the body's constitution (prakriti), and life forces (doshas) are the primary basis of ayurvedic medicine. Goals of treatment aid the person by eliminating impurities, reducing symptoms, increasing resistance to disease, reducing worry, and increasing harmony in life."

The key to bettering our physical and mental health lies in the concept of *doshas*. *Doshas* are our life force, our connection to the earth and the elements within it. How these two things work in tandem to keep us healthy. If we neglect the needs of one, then we're also neglecting the needs of the other. However, what makes taking proper care of yourself complicated comes from the fact that everyone has their own individual needs.

The main theme in Ayurveda is the idea that everyone is composed of the *Panchamahabhuta*, also known as the five great elements: Vayu (air), Teja (fire), Prithvi (earth), Jala (water), and Aakash (ether/space). These elements are said to comprise all living things, from the modern-day human to the budding sapling. However, certain individuals have higher concentrations of one element than they might have with another. When these dominant elements combine with us, they create a distinct blueprint that is known as our *dosha*. There are three main types of *dosha*: Vata, Pitta, and Kapha. Each is responsible for our mental, spiritual, and physiological balance. These *doshas* are a combination of elements that dictate a person's personality, temperament, and constitution.

Vata

The vata dosha revolves around the elements of air and ether/space. Air encompasses wind, steam, smoke: anything that can be considered a gas. Ether, or space, is a little more complicated though. According to Yoga Journal, "Space is the mother of the other elements. The experience of space as luminous emptiness is the basis of higher spiritual experiences." Both of these elements can be considered weightless, untethered to the world below. For that reason, vata is considered to be a force of mobility for the human body. It is the ability for us to move freely—like the air—and our potential for endless possibilities—like the ether.

People with the vata dosha are said to embody that sentiment, having an excess of enthusiasm and creativity. They're extremely flexible and skilled multitaskers, capable of scattering themselves over a variety of projects and finding various opportunities. However, their connection to these untethered elements also gives them the negative attributes of being easily distracted and forgetful. According to Yoga Journal, "The influence of the air element in their constitution causes their energy, mood, and appetite to fluctuate dramatically." When people are dominated by these boundless elements, it's hard for them to find a form of consistency.

Pitta

The pitta dosha revolves around water and fire. Water is a vast component of our bodies, human beings being on average 70% water. Within the body, water refers to saliva, urine, semen, blood, and sweat—according to Yoga Journal. Each of these fluids are vital to our wellbeing and the continuation of our species. Consistency is what the element of water embodies, the flow of a stream capable of eroding earth and rock. The element of fire, on the other hand, is a dynamic force capable of bringing change. It has the ability to both create and destroy: the burning of wood leading to the creation of smoke and ash. It is a tool that humans have used to better how we eat, how we build, and how we live.

While there is importance in both fire and water, one would be right in making the assumption that these two elements seem to counteract each other. The elements of fire and water are constantly at odds with each other, each fighting for dominance. It's the conflicting nature of these elements that makes those with this dosha naturally powerful people. These people embody the attributes of both water and fire; having the drive to achieve their goals as well as the resolve to stick with them. They are often the type to take charge, rather than take orders. However, the volatile nature of their elements often causes them to be aggressive and impatient. Their mood is quick to shift when things don't go their way, their combination of fire and water brawling within them.

Kapha

The kapha dosha revolves around water and earth. While water is a flowing and versatile element, the element of earth represents stability. According to Yoga Journal, "Earth is not just soil, but it is everything in nature that is solid." The snow-capped mountains and the deepest canyons have been around for millennia, and there are trees that have stood tall for hundreds of years. These two elements work together to nurture and foster life, and for that reason people with this dosha often function as a support system for others and try to maintain a balance amongst people. They have a sense of stability, having good control over their emotions. According to Healthline, "Kapha-dominant people rarely get upset, think before acting, and go through life in a slow, deliberate manner." However, this also tends to make them sluggish and less motivated. They also tend to feel depressed or anxious when changes are made or if they need to take risks. They're the kind of people to choose to take their time, rather than rush into things. Just as it takes decades for a tree to sprout from a sapling, it takes kapha-dominant people a considerable amount of time to find the urge to achieve their goals.

* * *

While there are three main doshas, it's possible for people to have more than one dosha. People who are considered bi-doshic (or even tri-doshic) have attributes that are linked towards more than one dosha. Combinations such as vata-pitta, pitta-kapha, and vata-kapha exist, so people can have a better understanding of how to care for themselves in a way that aids all their doshas.

SUBTLE FORMS

There is more to our selves than our inherent doshas. There are three subtle forms of these dosha that have an effect on our minds and bodies. Those forms are Prana, Tejas, and Ojas. These subtle forms can be found in the genetic make-up of every living being, encompassing several parts of our biology.

According to Easy Ayurveda, prana can be described as 'the life force' or 'the breath of life', making it a subtle form of the vata dosha. In terms of the body, this essence revolves around the respiratory system, blood circulation, digestion, basically any-thing that involves movement throughout the body. Mentally, it affects our impulses. Experiencing a decrease of prana means a person will suffer from a lack of motivation, also taking a hit in creativity, sociality, and receptivity.

Tejas, on the other hand, refers to the 'fire of the mind'. As one might assume, this essence basically deals with many factors of the mind. These include qualities such as intelligence, mental for-titude, perception, and inquisitiveness. It's the source of fervor, courage, and willpower within the human body. This means that it has a very close connection to the pitta dosha. Having a lack in this essence means you'll have a lack of focus, a lack of mental drive, and an increase of passivity. Having too much means you'll begin to feel an increase in irritability, anger, and doubt.

Ojas has to do with the 'primal vigor' inside a person, which mostly refers to the vital fluids found inside the body, as well as the tissues they aid. Blood, sweat, bile, and saliva are a few of the aspects that continually keep our bodies going. For this reason, it has a strong connection to the kapha dosha. According to Easy Ayurveda, "As per Yogic science, Ojas promotes mental strength, immunity, stability, endurance, patience, calmness, good memory, sustain concentration, happiness, contentment, and bliss. It connects our physical, mental, and spiritual well-being and peace of mind." Having lack of ojas means the person will be more likely to experience excess anxiety, a lack of concentration, and mental fatigue. Having too much means you'll experience a dullness of the mind or an unhealthy sense of complacency.

These three essences are present in everyone and are intertwined with one another. Much like most things in Ayurveda, how we tend to the needs of one reflects in the qualities of the others. Keeping in mind all these factors, a person will be able to sculpt their lives and schedules around what is best for their inner essences. In the words of Yoga International, "And since the combination of vata, pitta, and kapha are endless, each person has a constitution that is "as unique as his fingerprint."" Our bodies are unique to ourselves, and properly tending to our individual needs is key to living a healthy and happy lifestyle.

APPLYING THE PRACTICE TO OUR BODIES

While being able to know our dosha type is interesting—almost like having a separate horoscope—having that knowledge is only part of our journey into the practices of Ayurveda. How do we apply that knowledge so we may live healthier and ultimately happier lives? Now that we know what concepts Ayurveda touches upon, it's important for us to understand how we can use that information to improve our health and wellness. The link between our mind and body lies in the connection between a person's prakriti and dosha. The prakriti is a term that refers to a person's bodily constitution. This is closely linked to the person's dosha, which can have various effects on their health, both good and bad. Previously, we talked about the mental and emotional effects that a person's dosha can have, but now we'll move on to the effect it can have on a person's body.

However, how does a person know which dosha they fit under? In ancient India, the methods used to diagnose certain ailments in traditional ayurvedic treatments revolve around the study and observation of various aspects of the patient's health. These include Nadi (pulse), Mootra (urine), Mala (stool), Jihva (tongue), Shabdah (speech), Sparsha (touch), Druk (vision), and Aakruti (appearance). Most of these diagnoses require the practitioner to rely on their senses rather than the use of scientific instruments, such as checking the pallor of someone's skin or feeling a person's pulse. However, luckily for us living in the modern day, the internet makes it much easier to be able to get a feel for what your dosha type is. There are a number of quizzes online to help someone figure out where they stand in terms of dosha type.

THE 20 GUNAS

In Ayurveda, there are ten pairs of opposing qualities that our bodies can embody, depending on our individual dosha type. These attributes are known as the 20 gunas; depending on the gunas you have, you can classify yourself into a certain dosha type.

- Cold and Hot: The attributes hot and cold don't simply refer to the natural temperature of a person's body, but also to the effectiveness of a person's internal processes. The warmer the body, the more the body is working towards ensuring that the person is being kept healthy and well-nourished. A body that is considered cold may have a slower digestive system and reduced immunity, while a body that is hot would have better digestion and protection from diseases. That said, people with hot qualities are often prone to indigestion and inflammation as a result of their body's natural temperature.
- Light and Heavy: The attributes light and heavy don't necessarily have to do with a person's weight, but with a person's ability to grow from nutrients absorbed into the body. Someone with a light body has a constitution that doesn't promote much growth or natural stability, but they'll have better ease of movement than a naturally heavy person. A person with a heavy body has a

constitution that promotes an excess of growth, result-ing in more weight and less ease of movement. However, this also provides them with more stability and a better grounding force than someone with a light body.

- Dry and Oily: The attributes dry and oily are referring to the amount of moisture within a person's body. This moisture can be displayed in the skin, the lungs, and even the stool. Having a dry constitution means that your body has an absence of moisture, which can result in complications such as dry skin, constriction to the lungs, and constipation. People with an oily constitution may be spared from chapped lips and dry coughs, but they often experience an excess of oil clogging their bod-ies. This can result in acne flare ups and excess mucus within the lungs, throat, mouth and nose.

- Clear and Cloudy: The attributes clear and cloudy refer to the number of substances absorbed within the mind and body. Clearing out the body of toxins is essential to healthy living, but it's important not to go overboard. Someone with a clear constitution is said to have a relatively clean digestive system and healthy livers, but these people also have difficulty healing due to how bar-ren their systems are. Someone with a cloudy constitu-tion easily absorbs these external substances, bogging down their liver and digestive system. However, their approximation to those substances allows them to heal from broken bones and breakages in the skin faster.

- Subtle and Gross: The attributes subtle and gross have to do with the amount of blockages within a person's body. This doesn't simply have to do with the digestive sys-tem, but also the mind, such as excess stress or restless thoughts. A person with the subtle attribute is able to keep their bodies and minds free of these blockages, but in return they may feel a sense of spaciness or oversensi-tivity. Someone with the gross attribute may experience a lot of blockages in their life, both mentally and physically. They may struggle with their weight or have a hard time letting go of stress. However, these blockages aren't all bad, as they can give a person a sense of stability and realism.

- Mobile and Static: The attributes mobile and static have to do with a person's ease of movement, both inside and out. This may refer to the muscular systems, the digestive system, or even the mental flexibility of the brain. Someone who is more mobile is capable of moving quickly and being more adaptable to changes, but they may be restless and experience tremors and muscle spasms. Someone who is more static may be slower moving, as well as being prone to lethargy and blockages within the body. They may also be more fixed mentally, making it difficult for them to accept changes in their daily lives.

- Rough and Smooth: The attributes rough and smooth describe how a person absorbs moisture into their body. Someone with a rough body might have trouble absorbing moisture, leading to dryness, absorption, and constipation. These blockages can cause both the body and mind to be less flexible. Someone with a smooth body on the other hand may be more lubricated inside and out. This also tends to make their bodies and minds more flexible and helps to prevent arthritis and osteoporosis, according to Living Rasa. The downside of having this attribute is that having too much of it can lead to further oiliness and blockages within the body.

- Sharp and Dull: The attributes sharp and dull have to do with a person's ability to react to outside stimuli. Someone with a sharp body is capable of acting quickly, both in physical movement as well as their mental processes, capable of learning quickly and soaking up information like a sponge. However, this sharpness of mind and body also causes people with this attribute to suffer from excess stress, muscle spasms, and anxiety. Meanwhile, people with a dull body might be slower to react, giving them a sense of sluggishness and inertia, but this also means they're capable of retaining energy and fostering a feeling of calm within themselves.

- Hard and Soft: The attributes hard and soft have to do with the innate ability for the body to develop muscles and tissue to protect itself. Someone with a hard body may find it easy to build muscle and form hardened calluses over skin. However, this also works to their detriments as they'll be more likely to develop cysts and tumors. People with soft bodies may not have much muscle or definition, but their skin is naturally smooth and malleable. They also tend to have softer, more caring hearts than people who may have hardened themselves to the rest of the world.
- Dense and Porous: The attributes dense and porous (also known as solid and liquid) refer to the overall concentration of the body. This can be in regards to muscle, strength, cohesiveness and flexibility. Someone with a dense body is said to have a lot of healthy muscle and internal strength, but this also means they have very little room for change. They're said to have one-track minds, always focused on the task ahead. People with the porous attribute are less fixed in their mind and body. However, this makes them more flexible, their bodies able to move easier because of their less concentrated internal structures.

The elements within a single dosha type are characterized by many of these gunas. Each of these gunas can either increase or decrease a person's dosha. Depending on the type of gunas you have, you'll be able to figure out where you stand on the dosha spectrum, as well as figure out how to best take care of your body. The only way to aid your body's natural deficiencies is to decrease your dosha. In Ayurveda, "like increases like"; this means that the more you do things that fall in line with your dosha, the more you'll see that dosha's qualities within you. While this means that the good qualities provided by your dosha will be enhanced, that means the same thing for the negative qualities as well.

Vata

The vata dosha's connection to air and ether will give people with this dosha type similar attributes. People with the vata dosha type are characterized by having light, dry, and mobile bodies. They are often described as having lanky physiques, and some people have the tendency to become underweight. However, thin is not the only quality that a vata body type can have. According to Banyan Botanicals, the vata body type "may manifest as extremes; as in being very tall or very short or being drastically different weights at different times in your life."

Because of their untethered elements, consistency is something that vata-types struggle with, often being unable to commit to consistent healthy eating and exercise. The skin of people with the vata dosha is naturally coarse and dry, requiring constant moisture to retain a healthy sheen. They are also prone to experiencing circulation issues due to their naturally dry bodies, and some people report experiencing frequent heart palpitations. It's important for those with the vata dosha to schedule a regular, healthy routine. (No matter how difficult that may be for them.) This routine should consist of regular meals, daily exercise, and proper self-care to ensure that they are tending to the needs of their minds, bodies, and souls.

Pitta

The combination of water and fire may keep people with the pitta dosha type naturally moisturized, but it also makes their bodies naturally volatile. Those with the pitta dosha are said to have bodies characterized by hot, sharp, light, and oily qualities. The natural heat and moisture within them often has positive effects on their constitution. According to Banyan Botanicals, "The hot quality creates a healthy blush in the cheeks, a naturally strong digestive fire, the capacity to stay warm in cold conditions, and gives the personality passion." However, it's also important to remember that this hot and oily constitution can also have its downsides. This heat flushing to a person's complexion can lead to an excess of oil within the skin, leading to acne, rosacea, and other forms of skin inflammation. It also has the ability to spur acid reflux in the stomachs of people with this dosha type, as well as promoting irritability in their temperaments.

The most important thing for people with this dosha type to focus on is balance. These people are often so driven towards their goals that they neglect their own emotions, which can be a problem for both themselves and for others. It's important for them to balance work with self-care, tending to both their mental and emotional needs along the way.

Kapha

The Kapha dosha revolves around earth and water, elements that work in tandem to foster growth and prosperity. For that reason, their bodies are described as being static, dense, and oily. People with this dosha type have bodies that soak up nutrients like a sponge, retaining it for much longer than either the vata or pitta doshas. This gives them naturally moisturized skin and hair, as well as allowing them to reap the benefits from their healthy meals. However, this also means that they retain everything they eat for longer. The constant flow of nutrients and tepid digestive fire can lead to weight gain and lethargy. Some people even end up developing dangerous eating disorders such as anorexia and bulimia. Their skin is also unfortunately susceptible to water retention, causing swelling, puffy skin, and joint disorders.

In addition to these physical complications, people with the kapha dosha are also at risk of developing depressive disorders. The best thing that someone with this dosha type can do for their body is to focus on regular exercise and healthy eating. Since their bodies take longer to burn calories than people of the vata or pitta dosha type, it's important for them to both eat healthy and work on burning calories.

SEASONAL EFFECTS ON DOSHAS

While it's important to understand the internal factors that doshas have on our bodies, it's just as important to take into account the external factors as well. The elements around us can also have an effect on our overall health and mindset. These include the temperature outside, the weather, and most importantly, the current season. The doshas that we apply to our own bodies can also be used to classify the seasons. Seasons that are characterized by a certain dosha have an effect on our own personal doshas, either decreasing or increasing our dosha's attributes. It's important to not sculpt our routines around the inherent attributes displayed in our bodies, but also around the attributes displayed by nature itself.

Spring

The season of spring is something that has always been classified by several different cultures as a season of growth and rebirth. According to TripSavvy, "Vasant, or Basant, Panchami, marks the beginning of spring on the Hindu calendar and is considered an auspicious day for new beginnings such as starting a new business, getting married, holding a housewarming ceremony, or other important work." One of the most important of these new beginnings is the spring harvest, where farmers reap their rewards of a hard year's work. This season of growth and prosperity is why spring is considered a kapha season.

During the springtime, a person's kapha dosha increases, enhancing their good qualities while also worsening their bad ones. People with the kapha dosha may find that their skin is oilier than usual or they might find feeling more sluggish during this season. Their doshas can also be aggravated depending on the amount of rainfall their areas experience during the spring season. General advice for this kapha season would be to stay active and stay social. Much like spring fosters growth in the flora and fauna around us, it also promotes growth in our relationships. Physical activity can be used to counteract the natural heaviness of your dosha as well as the heaviness of the season.

Summer

Summer is a season characterized by heat and intensity. During these times, the world is hit with spikes of heat as people flock to the waters to keep cool. Beaches, lakes, pools all become more appealing to the masses as the temperature rises, and with the start of summer vacation many young people and their families are in dire need of some way to cool down. However, the summer season can also be a dangerous time for those near the water. When the hot front reaches the water, it collides with the cold air. This natural battle has the capacity to cause hurricanes, tornados, tsunamis, and violent storms capable of demolishing buildings and flooding towns. The overall heat and humidity of the season, as well as the storms that come with the summer months, is what fits it into the classification of a pitta season.

During this season, people with the pitta dosha may begin to see an imbalance in themselves, mirroring the imbalance of the summer season. They may notice a rise in irritability, they may experience acid reflux or heartburn, or they might be constantly aware of an uncomfortable heat within their bodies. In the words of Banyan Botanicals, "Your primary focus through the summer months will be to keep pitta balanced by staying cool, mellowing intensity with relaxation, and grounding your energy." Staying hydrated is key to surviving the heat and balancing out the volatility of your pitta dosha. They should also take the time to relax during their day, getting rid of some of that irritability, and remind themselves to take it slow.

Autumn

Autumn is a season characterized by change, the transition from the warmth of spring and summer to the shiver of winter. In the words of Banyan Botanicals, "Autumn harbors a certain emptiness that can leave us feeling exposed and a little raw, but it is also filled with possibility—a time when we, too, can strip down to a quiet essence of being and savor the simplicity." For that reason, autumn is considered a vata season.

This season doesn't only have a physical effect on people with the vata dosha, but also a psychological effect. The change that the season encapsulates, all while watching the world slowly wither around them, can give people with the vata dosha a sense of emptiness and disconnection from the rest of the world. In addition, they may begin to notice their skin growing dryer and more cracked or develop a dry cough from the moistureless air. It's important during this vata season to focus on keeping yourself warm and hydrated to combat the cool and dry temperatures. It's also important for you to keep your mind balanced as well, taking the time to quell any anxiety or stress that might come with the transition-based season. During this time, meditation can be a lifesaver for those dealing with restless thoughts. Keeping yourself healthy and centered in both body and mind is key to surviving a vata season.

Winter

After the fall ultimately comes winter, a season characterized by a deathly calm that comes over the world around us. The trees have lost their color, animals have begun their yearly hibernation, and whatever vegetation is left is slowly covered by freshly fallen snow. While many seasons can be traced to a single dosha, winter is a bit more complex, almost acting as a bi-doshic season. It's very strongly linked to the kapha dosha, but also has clear elements of vata within. "It is characterized by cold weather, a sense of heaviness, increased moisture (usually in the form of rain or snow), cloud-covered days, and the grounded, slow feeling that sends many animals into hibernation," according to Banyan Botanicals.

During this time, people might find themselves more hungry than usual. This is because a person's digestive fire words on overtime to regulate temperature and shield you from the cold. For that reason, it's important to stay warm and well-nourished during this season. Eating spicy foods or drinking hot beverages will not only satiate your stomach, but also help you keep a steady body temperature. Winter is also a good time to exercise and get your body moving; the spike in motion will bring your body temperature up and keep you warmer for longer.

❋ ❋ ❋

According to The Art of Living Retreat Center, there are three main categories to keep in mind when planning Ayurvedic treatments around the seasons. The Chaya seasons are meant for increasing your dosha, the Prakopa season aggravates your *doshas*, and the Prasama season pacifies your *dosha*. As an example, someone with the vata dosha might find their dry symptoms alleviated during a kapha month, but find them increased or aggravated during a vata month. It's important to keep these seasons in mind so that you know how to properly attend to the needs of your *dosha* during those times. That way you will always be able to tend to your own dosha's needs, depending on your current circumstances.

USING AYURVEDA TO CARE FOR OURSELVES

Now that we're aware of the various ways our dosha and the dosha around us can affect our bodies and minds, we can address the various ways we can tend to our individual needs through Ayurvedic treatments. As previously stated, Ayurveda is a lifestyle, meaning everything we do to take care of ourselves should be a daily routine that encompasses several aspects of our lives. This isn't something that you should do once and be done with. If you intend to follow the teaching of Ayurveda, this needs to be something you apply to our diets, our personal hygiene, our fitness regiment, and our methods of self-care.

Abhyanga Oil Massage

One of the major parts of the Ayurvedic lifestyle are the various massage practices surrounding it. Differentiating themselves from a regular massage you might get at the spa, "abhyanga, or oil massage, touts physical benefits like released muscle tension, lymphatic drainage, and more nourished skin from head to toe," in the words of the fashion magazine Elle. During the process of an abhyanga massage, the patient will have warm oil poured from head to toe onto their body, then have it slowly and methodically massaged into their skin. The purpose of an abhyanga is to relieve both the mind and body of internal stressors. This includes lowering blood pressure, relieving muscle stiffness, nourishing the skin, improving sleep, and alleviating anxiety. Abhyanga is appealing to many people because it doesn't necessarily need to be performed by a specialist. They can be done by the individual themselves. Self-massages are a good way for you to tend to your body without parting with a hefty sum of money to go to a massage therapist, all while being able to stay in the comfort of your own home.

It's important to remember that there is no one-size-fits-all in any Ayurvedic treatments. Depending on a person's dosha type (or dosha types) different methods will be used to attend to a person's body. In terms of abhyanga, the types of oils used differentiates from one dosha type to another. People with the vata dosha, due to their naturally cold and dry complexions, require oils that will raise their body's temperature and moisturize their skin. Oils such as sesame seed, almond, and avocado are recommended due to their warm and heavy attributes. Meanwhile, people with the pitta dosha require oils that are lighter, with a more cooling effect. Oils like this include coconut oil, sunflower oil, castor oil, and olive oil. People with the kapha dosha need something to counteract their heavy, cold body types. Warm, light oils such as flaxseed, corn, canola, and rosemary oil are great to raise their body heat and stimulate their senses.

If you chose to perform this massage on your own, it's important for you to remember not to rush. Slathering oils onto yourself for a few minutes isn't going to give you the desired results. It's not about moisturizing yourself and being done with it, it's about pampering yourself. In the Sanskrit language, the word *sneha* can be translated to both "love" and "oil". In the words of Chopra.com, "the effects of Abhyanga are similar to those received when one is saturated with love. Like the experience of being loved, Abhyanga can give a deep feeling of stability and warmth." This isn't only a matter of self-maintenance, but a form of self-care and an expression of self-love. At this moment, you are tending to yourself and only yourself, so it's important that when you perform this self-massage you are giving yourself the time and care you deserve.

Aromatherapy

Aromatherapy is another big part of Ayurvedic treatments. According to Sundari.com "aromas have a subtle, yet extremely powerful influence on our mind and body. Aromatherapy can be used to protect prana, regulate digestion and metabolism, and to boost immunity." When these fragrances are inhaled and received by our olfactory systems, it has a profound effect on the *prana* within the body, having the ability to influence a person's thoughts and emotions. Aromatherapy is often combined with various massage therapies to give the patient a sense of calm, relieving them of their tension and making the session a more tranquil experience. In Ayurveda, these aromas are meant to bring a balance to your dosha and alleviate some of the negative qualities that come with them.

As you can assume, different essential oils are used for aromatherapy depending on a person's dosha. The vata dosha is characterized by dryness and coldness. For that reason, people with this dosha type are recommended to use oils with warm, sweet aromas. These include scents like lavender, sandalwood, vanilla, cinnamon, and orange. The warmth of these scents quells the natural cold of vata-dominant people, and the heaviness of the sweeter scents counteracts the inherent lightness they possess. The pitta dosha on the other hand has more than enough heat to keep itself going. Therefore, people with the pitta dosha need a fragrance that will calm their turbulent bodies and minds. That's why it's recommended that they use fragrances that have a cooling effect on the body, such as jasmine, mint, chamomile, clary sage, and cypress. Meanwhile, the kapha dosha has a natural coldness and heaviness, so it's important for people with this dosha type to find warm, light fragrances to counteract those inherent attributes. Oils that can help to warm and stimulate the body include peppermint, rosemary, eucalyptus, and thyme. It's also possible to blend many of these oils, either to satisfy multiple doshas or to experience a more balancing effect on the mind, body, and soul.

Herbal Remedies

One of the best ways to ensure that you stay healthy is to prevent illnesses before they start. Herbal remedies were often used by Ayurveda practitioners to do just that. According to Verywell Health, "practitioners will generally use ayurvedic herbs to "cleanse" the body, boost defense against disease, and keep the mind, body, and spirit in balance." There are a variety of herbs used in these remedies, each having differing effects on a person's dosha type.

Ashwagandha is a very popular herb used in Ayurvedic treatments. This small shrub can be found in various places in the Middle East and Africa, and comes with its set of medicinal qualities. According to Healthline, "It's considered an adaptogen, which means that it's believed to help your body manage stress more effectively." Evidence has also been shown that it's capable of alleviating anxiety disorders and improving sleep patterns. This is a great herb to utilize if you're of the vata dosha type, since vata imbalances can cause excess stress and anxiety. Other herbal remedies that may bring balance to the vata dosha include chamomile, fennel, saffron, and poppy seeds.

The resin from the *Boswellia serrata* tree has been a part of Asian and African traditional medicine for centuries. Scientific studies have proven boswellia's curative abilities to reduce inflammation.

"Practitioners believe that these properties can aid in the treatment of chronic inflammatory conditions, such as asthma, cardiovascular disease, COPD, and ulcerative colitis," according to Verywell Health. This makes the so-called Indian frankincense a great choice for those of the pitta dosha, as imbalances in this dosha type can lead to rashes and inflammation of the joints, and can worsen pre existing conditions such as rheumatoid arthritis and heartburn. Other ingredients such as turmeric, cumin seeds, coriander, and mint can also be used to bring balance to the pitta dosha.

Asiatic pennywort, also known as gotu kola, is a leafy plant often used in Asian cuisine and traditional medicine. According to Verywell Health, "Gotu kola is believed by alternative practitioners to have antimicrobial, antidiabetic, anti-inflammatory, antidepressant, and memory-enhancing properties." This herb is often turned into a tonic to treat a variety of ailments, both physical and mental. There is evidence that it has the capacity to aid memory, alleviate symptoms of depression and chronic fatigue. For that reason, it's a great herbal remedy for kapha-dominant people, since imbalances in the kapha dosha include lethargy, depression, and a lack of motivation. Other ingredients that are good for the kapha dosha include ginger, cardamon, peppermint, ginseng, and cinnamon.

Facials

How we take care of our faces often has a direct link to how we view ourselves. When we're able to be comfortable in our own skin, our inherent beauty is able to shine through. For that reason, proper care of our faces is critical to how we carry ourselves as a whole. Any form of Ayurvedic facial is an herbal treatment that works to treat any skin related issues that you may have. According to The Ayurveda Experience, "The root of skin problems could be due to an aggravated dosha." So in order to combat these issues, it's important to use oils and cleansers that are going to pacify your personal dosha.

The number one problem that people with the vata dosha find with their faces is an overall lack of moisture. Chapped, cracked, and overly-sensitive skin is common for people of this dosha type. However, they're also more susceptible to the effect of aging. People with a vata imbalance are more likely to develop wrinkles earlier in their lifetime. The number one goal for this skin type is to keep the skin moisturized and well-nourished. According to Heidi Kinney, a practitioner at the Ayurvedic spa Pratima, vata skin "needs to be nourished with oils, and people with vata skin need to keep hydrated internally as well as externally to keep the skin from premature fine lines and loss of elasticity." Adding essential oils, such as sesame oil or jasmine oil, to your skincare regime is a great way to hydrate and alleviate dry skin. If you use facial scrubs, it might be a good idea to look for recipes with oatmeal or ashwagandha to reduce dryness and add more lustre to your complexion.

Because of the volatile nature of their natural complexion, people with the pitta dosha often suffer from various forms of skin irritation. These include but are not limited to acne, rosacea, dark spots, and sunburn. It's important for people with this dosha type to stay out of the heat, as the rising temperatures often causes these skin conditions to get worse. It's also important to use substances on your face that will have a cooling effect on your skin. Aloe vera, sandalwood, and coconut oil are great for pitta-dominant people because of their ability to reduce inflammation and get rid of excess oils within the skin. When making a facial scrub, ingredients like turmeric or chickpea flour are recommended because of their ability to soothe skin and to reduce the risk of inflammation.

Kapha skin is characterized as having an excess in moisture, which leads to excessive oiliness of the skin. Imbalances in the kapha dosha are often reflected in the skin by the development of pimples, whiteheads, blackheads, and boils. The number one goal of kapha-dominant people is to keep their skin clean and free of excess oils. For that reason, oil-based creams are something they should avoid. Instead, they should use lighter substances such as lavender, geranium, and eucalyptus to clean their skin. These oils have a detoxing effect on your pores, clearing out your system as well as stimulating the skin. When making a facial scrub, it's important to use lighter substances like turmeric, chickpea flour, or french green clay, which are able to clean out the skin without bogging it down with more moisture.

Diets

The saying "you are what you eat" is a phrase that has been around for decades, and nothing could be closer to the truth. Science has proven that how we provide our bodies with nutrients has a direct effect on us physically, mentally, and emotionally. This is a sentiment strongly illustrated in Ayurvedic practices. Our digestive systems, much like everything else in our bodies, are subject to these same rules. Changing our diet is one of the ways we can balance out our personal dosha and bring harmony to the entirety of ourselves. Keeping to this new dietary regimen will insure that we'll continue to live happy and healthy lives.

We know that the vata dosha encompasses the qualities of dryness, lightness, and coldness, but what does that mean in terms of our body? Well, the problem therein is that people with this dosha type often have an excess of air in their system, especially in their digestive tract. Having imbalances in the vata dosha can result in bloating, gas, constipation, and weight loss. For vata-dominant people, it is important for them to eat foods that are warm, moist, and nourishing to combat the usual dryness and coldness of their body's usual constitution. It's a good idea for them to incorporate more warm foods into their diets, as well as vata-pacifying foods like red lentils, sweet potatoes, pistachios, and wild rice. It's also important that they incorporate more hot or lukewarm drinks into their diets. Cold drinks will increase the cold qualities within the vata dosha type. Cooking food with oils, such as olive or coconut oil, will also help to dispels some of the inherent dryness of this dosha type.

The digestive system of a pitta dosha is more unstable, due to its connection with water and fire. If a person has too much of a pitta imbalance, it can cause symptoms like indigestion, heartburn, loose stool, and acid reflux. So dealing with the pitta dosha type, it's important to structure your diet around cooler, dryer, and denser foods that will soothe the body and reduce inflammation. Pitta-dominant people should favor foods like cabbage, pasta, mung beans, and kale to pacify their turbulent dosha type. These foods have a mild flavor and a cooling effect on the body, bringing a sense of calm to your normally turbulent digestive system. Eating raw fruits and vegetables as a snack is also a good way to keep your body cool and satisfied. It's also important that pitta-dominant people stay away from alcohol and caffeine, since these substances have a warming effect on the body.

For people of the kapha dosha, they don't have trouble keeping nutrients in their bodies. For that reason, their bodies are classified as heavy and heavy, and these qualities can also be seen in their digestive systems. People with a kapha imbalance often complain of indigestion, diarrhea, constipation, and lethargy. In order to prevent these symptoms, people with this dosha type should favor light and airy foods. These include black beans, spinach, berries, and sprouts. They should also avoid oily or moist foods such as dairy products, melons, and fried eggs. Eating meals containing spices like paprika, cumin, and garlic also help to pacify the traits of the kapha dosha. As for drinks, it's important for you to incorporate warm beverages into your diet, such as various teas (preferably without cream). Following this diet will help to settle the stomach and prevent lethargy and fatigue.

Yoga

What once started as a strictly spiritual practice rooted in Hinduism, yoga has become one of the most popular health movements in the modern day. Whether you believe the Vedic teachings or not, the fact is yoga is not only a great method for exercising, but it's also a great method of centering your mind. Yoga combines aspects of deep breathing and meditation with physical movement, leaving the person feeling both relaxed and invigorated after their session is done. According to Yoga Outlet, "The path of yoga seeks to unite body, mind, and spirit through meditation, breath work, philosophy, physical movement, and behavior principles." This holistic view of physical and spiritual health puts the teachings of yoga in line with the teachings of Ayurveda. When creating a yoga routine, it's important not only to keep in mind a certain dosha's *prakriti*, but also the inherent traits that come with it.

People with the vata dosha are very focused on movement. Their adherence to the elements of air and ether gives them a tendency to dart from one subject to another, always needing to be in constant motion. Unfortunately, this restless nature is often their downfall. According to Patricia Bohlen, osteopath and ayurvedic massage therapist, "Vatas are more likely to develop conditions such as anxiety, joint and back pain, and conditions of the nervous system." While it may seem more natural for people with the vata dosha to go for more dynamic poses, we need to remember that "like increases like." It's important for vata-dominant people to go against their natural inclination to fast and constant movement, and instead incorporate slower, more deliberate poses into their routine. These poses should focus on core strength to keep them grounded and more focused; good examples of this are mountain pose, staff pose, and tree pose. It's also a good idea to give yourself more resting poses so you can focus on deep breathing and meditation during your routine.

Pitta-dominant people on the other hand are characterized by transition and mutability. The elements of fire and water within them make them naturally passionate and enthusiastic. However the turbulent nature of their dosha also tends to give them problems controlling their anger and keeping their aggressive temperament in check. In order to soothe their naturally tumultuous personalities, it's important for pitta-dominant people to incorporate poses into their yoga routine that are capable of balancing their water and fire elements. According to Yoga Outlet, "Poses that compress the solar plexus and those that open the chest can be particularly beneficial. Pitta people should avoid or limit poses and styles that create too much warmth, such as Bikram Yoga." It's also a good idea to utilize poses that stretch out the spine. These poses often have a heart-opening effect, meaning they increase the circulation, expand the thoracic cavity, and open up the lungs. Heart-opening poses such as Camel, Bridge, and Floor Bow are a great way for pitta-dominant people to increase their circulation and balance out their dosha's elements.

The kapha dosha is built on stability, growth, and consistency. An imbalance in this dosha means they'll begin to experience a lack of motivation, as well as start to develop a more fixed mindset. The best way to combat the effects of kapha imbalance is to go against the inflexible nature of this dosha type. When structuring a yoga routine around the kapha dosha, one should incorporate poses that revolve around balance, agility, and movement. According to Bohlen, "Postures (also called asanas) for Kapha will strengthen the lungs, respiratory system and mobilize the internal organs. Asanas will be uplifting, activating and warming to increase energy and vitality." Poses such as Sun Salutations, Half Moon, and Triangle inspire movement within the body and stimulate the internal processes within it.

* * *

No matter what dosha you have or what methods you use to alleviate your inherent traits, the most important factor of any of these Ayurvedic treatments is balance. By keeping track of how you eat, how you exercise, and how to care for your body, you are making an effort to balance various elements in your life. However, it's not just about making small changes. We can't simply change one thing in our lives and expect that to give us the change we want to see. It needs to be a constant routine that we use to keep our minds, bodies, and spirits healthy.

AFTERWORD

Society has come a long way in terms of medicine. From herbal remedies to chemotherapy, over the years our understanding of the human body has only increased, allowing us to better care for ourselves and our loved ones. However, it is those first accounts of traditional medicine that created the foundation of what we have today. From the beginning of human civilization, people have used elements found in nature to alleviate the adverse symptoms of a variety of diseases. This ancient method is something we use even today. Our modern doctors and physical therapists have built their treatments off the foundation of those early healers.

Whether you believe in the practices of Ayurveda or not, it's clear that having a holistic approach to your health and wellness will only benefit you as a person. The internal stressors within the body have a direct effect on how we function as people. At the end of the day, by utilizing Ayurvedic treatments in our everyday lives we're not simply conforming to a certain belief system. We are tending to the needs of our mind, body, and soul in order to ensure we feel better throughout our everyday lives. It's through the concepts explored in Ayurveda that we as people will be able to feel healthy both inside and out.